MW01291848

ABG'S Made Easy

An Easy Reference for RN's and RRT's

By Damon Wiseley B.H.S.c., RRT

https://www.rtboardexamprep.com

https://www.respiratorytherapyprograms.com

ABG'S Made Easy

An Easy Reference for RN's and RRT's

Table of Contents

Introduction

About This Book

Congratulations on purchasing this book and beginning your journey to a better understanding of arterial blood gases! The work you do is vitally important to your patients' health and happiness, and I commend you on striving to be the best you can be!

Correct analysis of arterial blood gas results is vital to the diagnosis and management of patients with oxygenation and acid-base disorders.

However, recent clinical surveys have found:

"29% of ER doctors and 31% of critical care nurses were unable to correctly interpret ABGs."

In addition, studies assessing the impact of ABG misinterpretations have shown errors in patient management occurred in 33% of the patients studied.

Therefore, understanding when and why we order ABG's, how to classify the ABG, and how to interpret the results, is important to both your career and your patient's health.

So what makes this a good ABG book"? When I think of all the books out there on this subject, most of them are either too simplistic or way to complicated. None have yet to hit the target of being simple, correct, and useful in your daily work. Knowing the who, what, when, where and why questions regarding ABG's will arm you with all the useful information you need.

In all honesty, some material in this book is a bit complicated and may seem intimidating at first. That is just the brutal reality we all have to face when trying to learn something hard.

However, my goal is to break all this information down into simple language.

ABG FAQ

What are the indications for arterial blood gas analysis?
Indications for ABG testing are a matter of debate among health care professionals. In fact, these indications can vary a great deal among different hospitals and even among different doctors within the same hospital.

Here are general guidelines to help you choose when an ABG may be indicated.

1. To Help establish a diagnosis
2. To Guide ventilator management
3. Post ventilator changes
4. Dyspnea
5. Cyanosis
6. Neurological deterioration

What are contraindications to arterial blood gas analysis?
Sites that have failed the modified Allens test (choose another site)
Sites with severe peripheral vascular disease
Sites with distorted anatomy or malformations
Sites with local infection
Sites with arteriovenous fistulas or grafts
Sites with indwelling radial or brachial dialysis shunts
Patients with severe coagulopathy

What is the modified Allens test?
The Allens test is performed before puncturing the radial artery. This test ensures there will still be circulation to the patient's hand through the ulnar artery if the radial artery spasms or develops a thrombus, following puncture.

This collateral circulation to the hand from the radial and ulnar arteries, makes the radial artery the first choice for arterial puncture.

What does an ABG tell me?

Arterial blood gas analysis assesses a patient's acid-base status and adequacy of ventilation and oxygenation. Many disease states can alter the patient's acid-base status. For example, kidney failure or diarrhea can cause a *metabolic* acidosis. Respiratory failure and/or heart failure may lead to a *respiratory* acidosis.

Why is it important to maintain a normal acid-base status?

Some medications do not function well in an acidotic environment.
Acid-base imbalances can alter patients' electrolyte levels.

How do I interpret an arterial blood gas?

There are 6 basic questions to ask when interpreting an arterial blood gas. These questions will be covered in greater detail later in this book. However, these are the basic questions that must be answered when interpreting an ABG:

1. Is the pH acidemic or alkalemic?
2. Did the respiratory system, metabolic system, or both systems cause the disorder?
3. Is there partial or complete compensation of the pH?
4. If the ABG is a respiratory disorder, is it acute or chronic?
5. If there is a metabolic disorder, is the anion gap normal or elevated?
6. Is the patient hypoxemic and to what degree?

How do I know if the ABG is a respiratory disorder, metabolic disorder, or both?

Respiratory disorders are caused by carbon dioxide levels (PCO2) that become too high or too low. For example, if the PCO2 increases, the pH will decrease. This ABG will be classified as a respiratory acidosis, because the respiratory system (PCO2) caused the acidosis.

Metabolic disorders are caused by sodium bicarbonate levels (HCO3) that become too high or too low. For example, if the HCO3 decreases, the pH will decrease with it. This ABG would be classified as a metabolic acidosis, because the metabolic system (HCO3) caused the acidosis.

Respiratory & Metabolic disorders can occur at the same time. For example, a patient in respiratory and renal failure will have a mixed respiratory and metabolic acidosis.

What's the difference between acidemia and acidosis?
Acidemia refers to a low blood pH. Acidosis refers to the process that causes the low blood pH. The same applies to alkalemia and alkalosis.

What is type 1 respiratory failure?
Type 1 (hypoxemic) respiratory failure is the most common form of respiratory failure. Hypoxemic respiratory failure occurs when the PaO2 is less than 60 mm Hg in the presence of a normal or low PCO2.

What is type 2 respiratory failure?
Type 2 (hypercapnic) respiratory failure occurs when the PCO2 is greater than 50 mm Hg. Hypercapnic respiratory failure can be further subdivided into acute or chronic respiratory failure.

What ventilator changes can help correct a respiratory disorder?
Respiratory acidosis (uncompensated): Increase ventilation using the tidal volume or respiratory rate. Returning the PCO2 to normal in a patient with compensated respiratory acidosis is not advisable.

Respiratory alkalosis: Decreased ventilation using the tidal volume or respiratory rate.

Hypoxemia: Increase oxygenation with the FiO2 and/or PEEP. Other strategies include increasing the inspiratory time (be sure patient has enough time to exhale fully).

How long should I wait after changing a patient's oxygen level to draw a blood gas?
Wait at least 15 to 20 minutes for patients without lung disease. Wait 30 minutes for patients with lung disease. These

timeframes are general guidelines only and should only be used as guidelines and as tolerated by the patient.

I accidentally drew a venous sample; can I use any of the values?

The pH and HCO3 show similar results whether drawn from an artery or a vein. A recent study showed a mean deviation of just 0.03 units between samples for the pH (2014, Byrne et. al.). The HCO3 was shown to have a mean deviation of just 1.03 mmol/L

The PCO2 only correlates well between arterial and venous samples when the PCO2 is normal (2014, Byrne et. al.).

The PO2 does not correlate or compare well between arterial and venous samples.

How does a patient's temperature affect my sample results?

A hypothermic patient's ABG results will reveal a higher PaO2 and PCO2 than actual and a lower pH than actual, when not temperature corrected for the patient's actual temperature. Patients may be hypothermic following surgery, after a near drowning, or due to therapeutic hypothermia protocols for patients suffering from cardiac arrest.

Conversely, a hyperthermic patient's ABG will reveal a lower PaO2 and PCO2 than actual and a higher pH than actual, when not temperature corrected for the patient's actual temperature. Patients with fever or sepsis may be hyperthermic.

How do air bubbles in my sample affect the ABG results?

The PaO2 may be falsely higher or falsely lower, dependent upon if the patient is hypoxemic. Air bubbles in the sample will cause the PaO2 to move towards the PaO2 of room air, which is 150 mm Hg. This can cause a false high or a false low PaO2 reading, depending upon if the patient is hypoxemic.

If the patient *is* hypoxemic, the PO2 will appear falsely high as it increases to the PaO2 of room air. If the patient *is not* hypoxemic, the PaO2 will appear falsely low as it decreases to the PaO2 of room air.

An air bubble in the ABG sample will always cause the PCO2 to appear lower than it is. This is because there is essentially no carbon dioxide in room air.

How does liquid heparin affect my sample?

Liquid heparin has been shown to increase the PaO2 and decrease the PCO2 of ABG results. Liquid heparin's effect on the pH is minimal (Dake, et. al, 1984).

Sample dilution with liquid heparin may occur when drawing a sample from a heparinized arterial line or from an ABG syringe that contains liquid heparin, instead of dry heparin.

Do I need to place the sample on ice after drawing?

Different laboratories have different standards regarding when to place a sample on ice. However, a recent study revealed significant decreases in the pH and PaO2 and significant increases in PCO2 after only 15 minutes. These changes occurred in samples placed on ice, and samples left at room temperature (Srisan, P. et. al, 2011).

ABG Fundamentals

Acid-base Balance

Acid-base balance refers to the balance of acids and bases measured as pH. An acid-base disturbance occurs when the pH is shifted outside of its normal range of 7.35 to 7.45. Too much acid in the blood is acidemia. Too much base in the blood is alkalemia. These disturbances are then classified according to the cause of the imbalance (respiratory or metabolic) and the process occurring (acidosis or alkalosis).

PH

The abbreviation pH is derived from the phrase "**p**ower of **H**ydrogen." The H is capitalized, because it is an element. The pH of blood (or any water based solution) is a measure of its hydrogen ion concentration ($H+$).

The hydrogen ion concentration is inversely related to the pH level, meaning if one is high, the other is low and vice versa.

For example, a low concentration of hydrogen ions corresponds to a high pH. A high concentration of hydrogen ions corresponds to a low pH.

HCO3-

This calculated value represents the bicarbonate anion in arterial blood. 90% of carbon dioxide in the blood exists as $HCO3$.

BE

This calculated value represents the amount of base in the sample. A base excess occurs when there is excess base in the sample. A base deficit occurs when there is a deficit of base in the sample.

Ventilation & Oxygenation

Ventilation

Ventilation is the movement of air into and out of the lungs and is reflected by the PCO2. PCO2 is the partial pressure of carbon dioxide dissolved in the arterial blood.

When a patient cannot eliminate carbon dioxide (PCO2) fast enough, they develop a respiratory acidosis.

Oxygenation

The PaO2 and SaO2 reflect the patient's oxygen status.

The PaO2 is the partial pressure of dissolved oxygen in the arterial blood.

The SaO2 is the percentage of arterial blood saturated with oxygen.

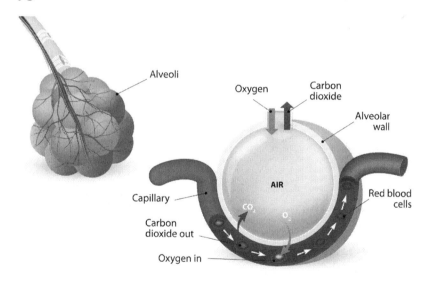

Oxy-hemoglobin dissociation curve

The Oxyhemoglobin dissociation curve provides a visual representation of how hemoglobin's affinity for oxygen changes due to changes in any of the following:

1. PH
2. Carbon dioxide
3. 2, 3 DPG (an organic phosphate produced by the red blood cells)
4. Body temperature

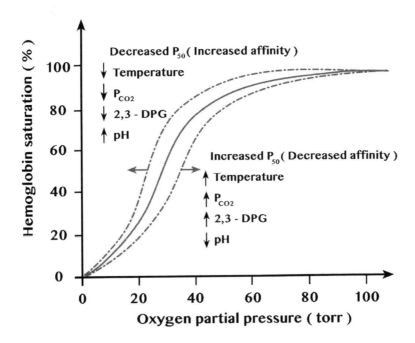

Left shift

A left shift means a lower PaO2 will be required to achieve the same saturation of hemoglobin as compared to no shift at all. A left shift increases hemoglobin's affinity for oxygen. The result is higher oxygen content relative to PO2. When the SaO2 reaches a high level, large increases in PO2 will result in only minor increases in SaO2.

Right shift

A right shift means a higher PaO2 will be required to achieve the same saturation of hemoglobin as compared to no shift at all. A right shift reduces hemoglobin's affinity for oxygen. This makes it easier for hemoglobin to release oxygen, but harder to bind with it. As a result, a right shift means a higher PO2 is required to achieve the same SaO2.

P50

P50=the PO2 at which hemoglobin is 50% saturated.

Normal ABG Values

Parameter	Normal Range
pH	7.35 – 7.45
PaCO2	35 – 45 torr
PaO2	80 – 100 torr
HCO3-	22 – 26 mEq/L
BE	-2 - +2 mEq/L
SaO2	95 – 100%
CaO2	12 – 16 Vol%

Acid-Base Disturbances

Respiratory Acidosis

Respiratory acidosis occurs when more carbon dioxide is produced than can be eliminated through respiration. Respiratory acidosis may also be referred to as respiratory or ventilatory failure.

Respiratory acidosis may be classified as acute or chronic. Acute respiratory acidosis occurs abruptly. Chronic respiratory acidosis occurs over an extended period of time and is accompanied by partial or complete renal compensation of the pH.

Acute respiratory acidosis

PH	PCO2	HCO3
Low	High	Normal

Chronic respiratory acidosis (fully compensated pH)

PH	PCO2	HCO3
Normal	High	High

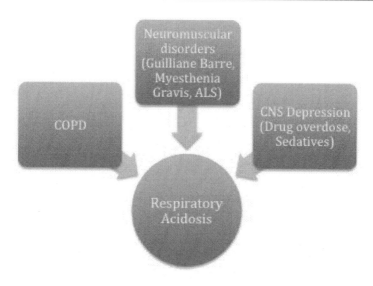

Respiratory Alkalosis

Respiratory alkalosis occurs when too much carbon dioxide is removed from the body as a result of hyperventilation.

PH	PCO2	HCO3
High	Low	Normal

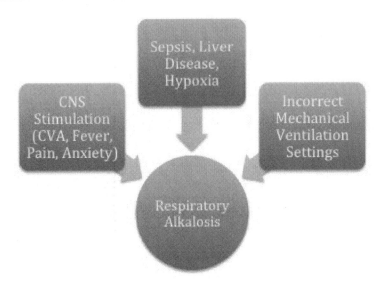

Metabolic Acidosis

Metabolic acidosis occurs when the body produces or retains too much acid. This leads to an acidemic pH, which results in metabolic acidosis. Anion gap calculation helps differentiate the type of metabolic acidosis. Calculate the anion gap to help determine the cause of the acidosis.

PH	PCO2	HCO3
Low	Normal to Low	Low

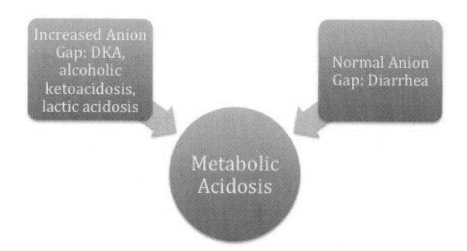

Metabolic Alkalosis

Metabolic alkalosis occurs when the body loses too many hydrogen ions or gains too much HCO3-.

PH	PCO2	HCO3
High	Normal	High

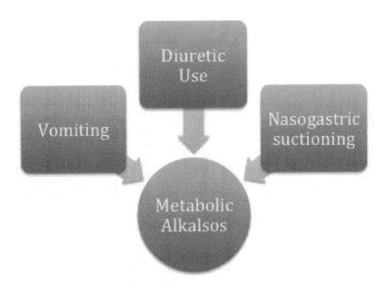

ABG Interpretation

Correctly analyzing and interpreting an arterial blood gas involves many steps. However, the most important step is performed before the test is even performed. This important step is to identify the acid-base disorder you suspect based on the patient's history, signs, and symptoms. After deciding on possible acid-base disturbances, the following steps must be performed to interpret the ABG.

Step 1: Is the pH acidemic or alkalemic?

Acidemia	Normal	Alkalemia
pH <7.35	pH 7.35 to 7.45	pH >7.45

Step 2: Did the respiratory system (PCO2), metabolic system (HCO3), or both systems cause the disturbance?

Acid-base disturbance

Respiratory Acidosis	HCO3 Normal	↑ PCO2
Respiratory Alkalosis	HCO3 Normal	↓ PCO2
Metabolic Acidosis	↓ HCO3-	PCO2 Normal
Metabolic Alkalosis	↑HCO3-	PCO2 Normal
Respiratory & Metabolic Acidosis	↓ HCO3-	↓ PCO2
Respiratory & Metabolic Alkalosis	↑HCO3-	↑ PCO2

Step 3: Is there partial or complete compensation of the pH? Compensation is the body's effort to maintain homeostasis by returning the pH to normal.

Renal compensation of respiratory disorders is a slow process that can take 3 to 5 days to complete. By contrast, respiratory compensation of metabolic disorders begins immediately by increasing alveolar ventilation.

Acid-base disorder	Compensatory Response
Respiratory Acidosis	Kidneys hold on to HCO_3-
Respiratory Alkalosis	Kidneys dump HCO_3-
Metabolic Acidosis	Ventilation increases to decrease PCO_2
Metabolic Alkalosis	Ventilation decreases to increase PCO_2

Partial compensation occurs when the compensatory response does not change the pH to normal.

Full compensation occurs when the compensatory response returns the pH to normal.

Note: Classic studies regarding complete compensation of the pH have suggested it is near impossible to return the pH back to normal. However, these studies were performed on canines and contradict routine observations of complete compensation of chronic respiratory acidosis in the human population (Martinu, T. et. al., 2003).

Step 4
Respiratory disorders may also be described as acute or chronic.

Acute Respiratory Disorder

Acute changes in PCO2 have a profound effect on the pH before the slow process of renal compensation occurs. As a result, an acute respiratory disorder will reveal little to no compensation.

For every 10 mm Hg shift in the PCO2, the pH will shift 0.08 units during an acute respiratory disorder.

Change in PCO2	Expected pH change: Acute disorder
↑ PCO2 by 10	↓ pH by 0.08 units
↓ PCO2 by 10	↑ pH by 0.08 units

Chronic Respiratory Disorder

After 3 to 5 days, renal compensation of the acute respiratory disorder will diminish the PCO2's effect on the pH. For every 10 mm Hg change in PCO2, the pH will shift only 0.03 units during a chronic respiratory disorder.

Change in PCO2	Expected pH change: Chronic disorder
↑ PCO2 by 10	↓ pH by 0.03 units
↓ PCO2 by 10	↑ pH by 0.03 units

Step 5

If a metabolic disorder exists, calculate the anion gap. The anion gap represents the difference between cations (positively charged ions) and anions (negatively charged ions) in the blood. Calculating the anion gap helps distinguish an anion gap metabolic acidosis from a non-anion gap metabolic acidosis. This helps narrow down the possible causes of the metabolic acidosis.

To calculate the anion gap, you will need a chemistry panel that includes the sodium, and chloride values.

The anion gap = Sodium – (Chloride + Bicarbonate)

Normal anion gap = 8 to 12

Anion gap metabolic acidosis causes
Methanol intoxication
Uremia
Diabetic or alcoholic ketoacidosis
Paraldehyde
Isoniazid or **I**ron overdose
Lactic acid
Ethylene glycol intoxication
Salicylate intoxication

Non-anion gap metabolic acidosis causes
Diarrhea
Gastrointestinal fistula
Renal tubular acidosis

Step 6: Assess oxygenation
First, look at the PaO2 to determine if the patient is hypoxemic.

Hypoxemia

Mild	PaO2 60 – 79 mm Hg
Moderate	PaO2 40 – 59 mm Hg
Severe	PaO2 < 40 mm Hg

Next, calculate the A-a gradient if the patient meets any of the following conditions:

1. The patient is hypoxemic.
2. The patient is on oxygen.
3. The patient is hyperventilating.

Calculating the A-a gradient helps distinguish between intrapulmonary (pulmonary edema, pneumonia) and extra-pulmonary (anemia, sleep apnea) causes of hypoxemia.

A-a gradient formula: (150 - PaCO2/0.8) - PaO2

Practice Question
What is the A-a gradient for a patient with a PCO2 of 40, and a PO2 of 80?

Answer
First divide the PCO2 by 0.8	40/0.8 = 50
Next subtract 50 from 150	150 – 50 = 100
Then subtract the PaO2 from 100	100 – 80 = 20

Normal A-a gradient causes	Elevated A-a gradient causes
Hypoventilation	Diffusion defect
High altitude	Ventilation/perfusion mismatch
	Right to left shunt

A normal A-a gradient should be less than the patient's age (divided by 4) plus 4.

Practice Question
Find the normal A-a gradient for a 60-year-old patient.

Answer
Divide the patient's age by 4	60/4 = 15
Then add 4	15 + 4 = 19

The normal A-a gradient for a 60-year-old patient is less than 19.

ABG Collection

What are potential complications of arterial puncture?
1. Bleeding
2. Nerve damage
3. Vessel spasm
4. Thrombosis
5. Hematoma

What sampling errors can affect ABG results?

Errors affecting the accuracy of arterial blood gas results can occur before, during, or after the sample is drawn. However, pre-analytical errors account for 75% of errors during arterial blood gas analysis (Ancy, J., 2012).

1. Inadequate mixing prior to analysis
2. Sample dilution from arterial line flush solutions
3. Sample hemolysis, clotting
4. Air bubbles within the sample
5. Venous blood mixing into arterial sample during puncture
6. Delayed analysis greater than 15 minutes

How do I choose which site to draw the ABG from?

ABG's are drawn by directly puncturing the artery, or from an indwelling catheter such as an arterial line. If there is no arterial line, the first choice is the radial artery, followed by the brachial and femoral arteries.

Radial artery

Advantages
1. Collateral circulation
2. Close to skin surface
3. Easy to locate and palpate
4. Easy access from the bedside

Several factors make the radial artery the first choice for arterial puncture. First and foremost, the radial and ulnar artery provides collateral circulation to the hand. As a result, if the radial artery were damaged, blood would still flow to the hand. Should the brachial or femoral arteries sustain vessel damage, the appendage supplied with blood from that artery would be at risk of ischemia.

Brachial artery
The brachial artery does not provide collateral circulation downstream.

Femoral artery
The femoral artery does not provide collateral circulation downstream from the puncture site.

How do I perform the modified Allen's test?
Prior to attempting arterial puncture of the radial artery, a modified Allen's test may be performed to ensure there is collateral blood flow to the hand. This test is not technically considered a standard of care, however, it can be helpful in certain patient populations such as those considered high risk of arterial thrombosis.

Procedure
1). Have the patient make a clenched fist
2). Compress the patient's ulnar and radial artery to stop blood flow to the hand
3). Have the patient open and relax their hand (the hand should be blanched white).
4). Release pressure over the ulnar artery and observe the time it takes for color to return.

Normal color should return in 5 to 10 seconds indicating a positive or normal Allen's test. If color takes longer than 10 seconds consider another site. Currently debate exists regarding the usefulness of the Allen's test in predicting complications from ischemia.

Interpretation Practice

1. A patient with a history of severe diarrhea would most likely have which of the following acid-base disturbances?

    A. Metabolic alkalosis
    B. Metabolic acidosis
    C. Respiratory acidosis
    D. Respiratory alkalosis

2. A patient with a history of sever vomiting would most likely have which of the following acid-base disturbances?

    A. Metabolic alkalosis
    B. Metabolic acidosis
    C. Respiratory alkalosis
    D. Respiratory acidosis

3. A patient presents to the emergency room with a history of COPD, infiltrates in the right lower lobe, dyspnea and fever. The patient would most likely have which of the following acid-base disturbances?

    A. Compensated respiratory acidosis
    B. Uncompensated respiratory acidosis
    C. Metabolic alkalosis
    D. Metabolic acidosis

4. Classify the following ABG:
pH	7.37
PCO2	54
HCO3	32

    A. Compensated respiratory acidosis
    B. Partially compensated respiratory acidosis
    C. Metabolic acidosis
    D. Metabolic alkalosis

5. Classify the following ABG:

pH	7.32
PCO2	51
HCO3	24
PO2	58

   A. Respiratory acidosis with normal oxygenation
   B. Respiratory alkalosis with severe hypoxemia
   C. Respiratory acidosis with moderate hypoxemia
   D. Respiratory acidosis with severe hypoxemia

6. Classify the following ABG:

PH	7.30
PCO2	65
HCO3	24

   A. Respiratory alkalosis
   B. Respiratory acidosis
   C. Metabolic acidosis
   D. Metabolic alkalosis

7. Classify the following ABG:

PH	7.47
PCO2	32
HCO3	25

   A. Metabolic acidosis
   B. Metabolic alkalosis
   C. Combined respiratory & metabolic alkalosis
   D. Respiratory alkalosis

8. Classify the following ABG:

PH	7.32	Low
PCO2	54	High
HCO3	30	High

   A. Respiratory acidosis
   B. Respiratory & metabolic acidosis
   C. Partially compensated respiratory acidosis
   D. Metabolic alkalosis

9. Classify the following ABG:
   PH   7.37
   PCO2   58
   HCO3   32
   A. Compensated respiratory acidosis
   B. Acute respiratory acidosis
   C. Normal
   D. Respiratory & metabolic alkalosis

10. Classify the following ABG:
   PH   7.28
   PCO2   54
   HCO3   18
   A. Combined respiratory & metabolic acidosis
   B. Combined respiratory & metabolic alkalosis
   C. Metabolic alkalosis & metabolic acidosis
   D. Respiratory acidosis

11. What is the anion gap for a patient with the following lab values?
   Sodium = 120
   Chloride= 100
   Bicarbonate = 10
   A. 10
   B. 15
   C. 20
   D. 25

12. How should a PaO2 of 41 mm Hg be classified?
   A. Normal
   B. Mild hypoxemia
   C. Moderate hypoxemia
   D. Severe hypoxemia

13. What is the normal A-a gradient for a 40-year-old patient?
   A. Less than 23
   B. Less than 10

C. Less than 6

D. Less than 40

14. How much should the pH change for every 10 mm Hg change in PCO2 in a patient with acute respiratory acidosis?

    A. 0.03 units

    B. 0.06 units

    C. 0.09 units

    D. 0.08 units

15. How much should the pH change for every 10 mm Hg change in PCO2 in a patient with acute respiratory acidosis?

    A. 0.03 units

    B. 0.06 units

    C. 0.09 units

    D. 0.08 units

Answer Key

1. B, metabolic acidosis

2. A, metabolic alkalosis

3. B, uncompensated respiratory acidosis

4. A, compensated respiratory acidosis

5. C, respiratory acidosis with moderate hypoxemia

6. Respiratory acidosis.
   - The pH is acidemic
   - The low pH correlates with a high PCO2
   - There is no compensatory response yet from the kidneys, because the HCO3 is normal.

7. Respiratory alkalosis
   - The pH is alkalemic
   - The high pH correlates with a low PCO2
   - There is no compensatory response yet from the kidneys, because the HCO3 is normal.

8. Partially compensated respiratory acidosis
   - The pH is acidemic
   - The low pH correlates with the high PCO2. The low pH does not correlate with a high HCO3. Therefore, the ABG is a respiratory acidosis.
   - The HCO3 is partially compensating the pH by increasing above normal.

9. Compensated respiratory acidosis
   - The pH is normal, however, the PCO2 and HCO3 are both elevated.
   - The pH is on the low side of normal, which correlates with the high PCO2.

- The HCO3 has fully compensated the pH by raising it to the normal range.

10. Combined respiratory & metabolic acidosis
    - The pH is acidemic
    - Both the PCO2 *and* the HCO3 caused the acidemia.

11. A, The anion gap calculation is Sodium – (chloride + Bicarbonate). Plugging the numbers in we get 120 – (100 + 10) which = 10.

12. C. Moderate hypoxemia

13. C, less than 6. The normal A-a gradient for a 40 year old patient should be less than his age (divided by 4) + 4.

14. D, 0.08 units

15. A, 0.03 units

For more FREE tips, tricks, and courses designed to help you gain confidence with respiratory therapy topics, please visit:

http://www.respiratorytherapyprograms.com

https://www.rtboardexamprep.com

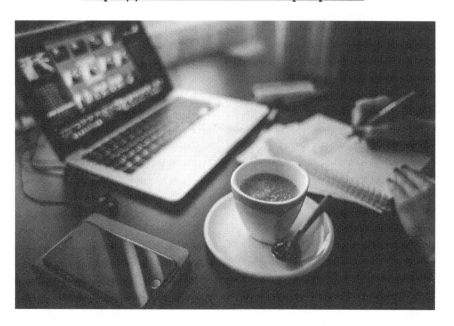

More By The Author

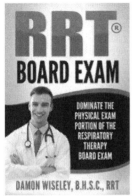

Available at: http://www.amazon.com/dp/B01BM0AK3S

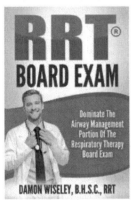

Available at: http://www.amazon.com/dp/B01DI71PU0

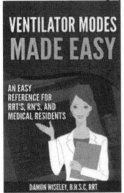

Available at: http://www.amazon.com/dp/B00P085K5C

References

Ancy J. Preventing preanalytical error in blood gas analysis (The blood gas laboratory) J Respir Care Sleep Med Spring. 2012;30:64.

Austin, K. and Jones, P. (2010), Accuracy of interpretation of arterial blood gases by emergency medicine doctors. *Emergency Medicine Australasia*, 22: 159–165. doi:10.1111/j.1742-6723.2010.01275.x

Bloom, B., Grundlingh, J., Bestwick, J., Harris, T.,(2014) The role of venous blood gas in the emergency department: a systematic review and meta-analysis. *European Journal of Emergency Medicine.* Apr;21(2):81-8. doi: 10.1097/MEJ.0b013e32836437cf.

Broughton, J., Kennedy, T., (1985). Interpretation of arterial blood gases by computer. *Chest.* 85: pg. 148-149.

Byrne A. L., Bennett M., Chatterji, R., Symons, R., Pace, N.L., Thomas, P.S., (2014), Peripheral venous and arterial blood gas analysis in adults: are they comparable? A systematic review and meta-analysis. Respirology. 19(2): pg. 168-175. Doi: 10.1111/resp.12225.

Dake, M., Peters, J., Teague, R., The effect of heparin dilution on arterial blood gas analysis. West J Med. 1984 May; 140(5): 792–793.

Doig, A., Albert, R., Syroid, N., Moon, S., Agutter, J. (2011), Graphical arterial blood gas visualization tool supports rapid and accurate data interpretation. *CIN: Computers, Informatics, Nursing*: April 2011 - Volume 29 - Issue 4 - pp 204-211 doi: 10.1097/NCN.0b013e3181fc4041

Kaynar, A. M., Pinsky, M. R., Aug 11, 2016. Respiratory Failure. *Medscape. Drugs & Diseases*

Martinu, T., Menzies, D., Dial, S., (2003). Re-evaluation of acid-base prediction rules in patients with chronic respiratory acidosis. *Canadian Respiratory Journal.* Sep;10(6):311-5.

Sood, P., Paul, G., & Puri, S. (2010). Interpretation of arterial blood gas. *Indian Journal of Critical Care Medicine* : Peer-Reviewed, Official Publication of Indian Society of Critical Care Medicine, 14(2), 57–64.

Srisan , P., Udomsri, T., Jetanachai, P., Lochindarat, S., Kanjanapattankul, W., (2011). Effects of temperature and time delay on arterial blood gas and electrolyte measurements. *Journal of the Medical Association of Thailand.* Aug;94 Suppl 3:S9-14.

Made in the USA
Columbia, SC
17 September 2024

42509086R00022